Christ Walk
Kids

Christ Walk
Kids

A 40-Day
Spiritual
Journey for
Tweens and Teens

ANNA FITCH COURIE

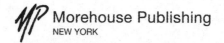 Morehouse Publishing
NEW YORK

All scripture quotations unless noted otherwise are taken from the Common English Bible, copyright 2011. Used by permission. All rights reserved.

Morehouse Publishing, 19 East 34th Street, New York, NY 10016

Morehouse Publishing is an imprint of Church Publishing Incorporated.
www.churchpublishing.org

Cover design by Laurie Klein Westhafer, Bounce Design
Typeset by Beth Oberholtzer

Library of Congress Cataloging-in-Publication Data
A record of this book is available from the Library of Congress.

ISBN-13: 978-0-8192-3319-6 (pbk.)
ISBN-13: 978-0-8192-3320-2 (ebook)

Printed in the United States of America

For Patton and Merryn. All my love.

Contents

A Letter to Parents

Christ Walk Kids covers many topics related to health and spirituality: physical exercise, nutrition, sex, drinking, drugs, praying, lying, stealing, bullying, and many others. I did not write this book for kids to read in a vacuum, but as though I were talking to my own children with the hope that it would open up honest dialogue between us. I hope you will also read the book with your children and go on a journey with them that helps to build a foundation of healthy choices for their minds, bodies, and spirits. Having an open dialogue about any subject with our children is the key to understanding what is going on in their brains and their lives. This book is how I talk to my kids; it may not be how you would talk to yours, so again, include yourself on their journey and share your own thoughts and feelings on the topic. You may be surprised at the discussion the topics generate. Be open; listen actively; and no matter what you hear, love your child anyway.

—Anna

Introduction

After the last ten years of being involved in the Christ Walk program, my children have had a natural curiosity with their mom being involved in the church and fitness. Both of them have read parts of the *Christ Walk* book at various times, but in all honesty, *Christ Walk* is for adults, not kids.

The way you speak to an adult is not the same way you would speak to a child. So at the request of my children, as well as several of my Christ Walk churches, I have put pen to paper, to distill Christ Walk into a book that focuses on our youth.

The goal of this book is to share with my children, you, or your children those things about mind, body, and spiritual health that are important as we grow and develop. Our children are inquisitive about their health, their bodies, their relationship with God, and their purpose in the world. It is my hope that *Christ Walk Kids* takes them on a journey towards mind, body, and spiritual health that will last them a lifetime.

—Anna

An Introduction to Christ Walk Kids

BIBLICAL BIG IDEA #1

And walk in love, as Christ loved us and gave himself up for us.
—Ephesians 5:2a (ESV)

You are going to take a journey over the next forty days. You are going to take this journey with yourself and with God. I want you to pick a Bible route from the list in Appendix A and commit to doing exercise that will add up to the miles of this journey.

Ask your mom, dad, or church to get you a fitness tracker (Fitbit, pedometer, Garmin Connect, or something similar). You will want to clip this to your pants or wrist to track the exercise you do each day. You can write your daily miles in this book and then add up all the miles of exercise you do for the next forty days to see how far you can go.

Why should you do this? Forty days is a powerful time in the Bible. It can also be a time for God to transform you as a Christian. The next forty days are all about making a covenant with God about taking care of your body. Your body is God's temple in the world and all the things you do with your body show God's love to other people.

In addition, it is fun. How far can you go? Can you get mom or dad to also track miles over the next forty days? Can you beat them? Can you beat your brother or sister if you have one? Put a chart on the refrigerator including everyone in the family to see how far we can go together on a walk with Christ the next forty days. We will talk each day about different things you can do to live a healthy life with God. It will be fun! Come on!

What do you need to do?

1. Get a fitness tracker.

2. Pick a Bible route from Appendix A to commit to walking, running, biking, swimming, dancing, or other activity.

3. Start exercising and tracking your miles.

4. Read about the Bible route you chose and think about what God was doing in the world on this journey.

5. Read a chapter a day for the next forty days and let us discuss what it means to be a Christ Walk Kid.

THINGS TO THINK ABOUT

1. What exercise do I want to commit to for the next forty days?

2. How can I get my mom, dad, siblings, a friend, or someone else involved?

3. What promise will I make to God the next forty days?

DAY 1 Steps taken: _____   Miles journeyed: _____

Exercise chosen: _____

What I told God today: _____

_____

_____

_____

_____

Something I thought about: _____

_____

_____

_____

_____

DAY 2
How Did God Make Me?

BIBLICAL BIG IDEA #2

God created humanity in God's own image, in the divine image God created them, male and female God created them.
—Genesis 1:27

God made boys and girls in God's image. We each have characteristics that reflect what God looks like. Each of us carries a little bit of Christ in us.

Instead we are God's accomplishment, created in Christ Jesus to do good things. God planned for these good things to be the way that we live our lives.
—Ephesians 2:10

Because we carry a little bit of Jesus in each of us, our job is to take care of the bodies that God gave us and use this body to do God's work in the world. When we use our bodies to do God's work in the world, we are reflecting the love of Jesus in each of us to everyone around us.

During Jesus' time on earth, people did not have cars, airplanes, trains, or other automatic transportation. They either walked or rode camels or donkeys. This is why during the forty days of Christ Walk Kids you are focusing on accomplishing a walking (or other fitness) goal. Think about the different journeys that people took during Jesus' time on foot. What do you think it would be like to be a part of that journey? Do you think it was hard to walk all the time? Do you think it would be exciting to be a part of Jesus' adventures?

Our bodies are special: They move, run, work, love, hug, hold hands, give high-fives, dance, play, and serve others. Your body should be special to you. You should take care of your body and treat it as though it is a gift from God (because it is).

THINGS TO THINK ABOUT

1. What do I think of my body?

2. How can I remember that a part of God is a part of my body?

3. What do I think of taking care of my body and doing God's work in the world?

DAY 2 Steps taken: _____ Miles journeyed: _____

Exercise chosen: _____

What I told God today: _____

_____

_____

_____

_____

Something I thought about: _____

_____

_____

_____

_____

DAY 3

What Can I Do With This Body?

BIBLICAL BIG IDEA #3
Go in peace. The LORD *is watching over you on this trip you've taken.* —Judges 18:6.

God calls us to take care of our bodies. Your body is the tool God has to make change in the world. God's word says we should honor our body.

Don't you know that your body is a temple of the Holy Spirit who is in you? Don't you know that you have the Holy Spirit from God, and you don't belong to yourselves? You have been bought and paid for, so honor God with your body. —1 Corinthians 6:19–20

Because God has given us such a cool tool to do work in the world, we need to take care of it just like any other tool. I'm talking about our bodies! This means we need to eat a variety of healthy foods, we need to exercise, we need to rest, and we need to laugh daily. When we have joy and happiness in our lives, we are able to share that joy and happiness with others. When we are taking care of our bodies by eating, sleeping, exercising, and finding joy each day then we are building a strong temple. This temple that is our body is then more able to do God's work in the world. That means you will be stronger, faster, and filled with more joy and energy to share with your friends, family, and community. When you take care of your body, you can do anything with it that God has called you to do.

You will be able to move mountains, serve meals, build houses, teach at schools, travel to far off lands, tend gardens, run races, write books, and share yourself and God with others. The possibilities are endless.

THINGS TO THINK ABOUT

1. What do I need to do to take care of my body?

2. How am I exercising, eating, sleeping, and finding joy each day?

3. What dreams do I have of doing great things with this body?

DAY 3 Steps taken: _____ Miles journeyed: _____

Exercise chosen: _____

What I told God today: _____

_____

_____

_____

_____

Something I thought about: _____

_____

_____

_____

_____

DAY 4
Where Can I Go With This Body?

BIBLICAL BIG IDEA #4

The land on which you have walked will forever be a legacy for you and your children. This is because you remained loyal to the LORD my God. —Joshua 14:9

What do you want to do with yourself? What are your dreams, hopes, or passions? What do you want to accomplish in this world? God gave you your body to do those things. You are only limited in where you go with your body by what you think you can do.

I was never an athlete. I was more on the arts and theater side of things when I was in school. I was active, but not an athlete. I think this is okay. We are all different. If there were only athletes in this world, then we would miss the great minds that create art, music, theater, dance, books, and more for the world to enjoy. There is a place for us all. God has a purpose for the artists, the athletes, the healers, the teachers, and all of us.

However, as I got older, and I went to work, I found that I really needed to find a sport or activity to keep me healthy. This made me take on something I had never done before: running. It was one of the most difficult tasks for me as an adult. You may laugh and think running is easy, but I will tell you, when you take on new things as you get older it is harder to learn them! Our bodies slow down and change in their ability to learn new things the older we get. This does not mean that we *cannot* learn new things, it just means the older you get, the harder it becomes. Today, you can learn almost effortlessly. You are learning daily. *This* is the time to find what you love (especially in physical exercise) and become really good at it.

Taking on new activities, new sports, and new hobbies means learning a discipline. You need to practice this discipline repeatedly for it to become a part of your daily life. Some new tasks may be difficult, but if you love it, and stick with it, it will become a habit for a lifetime.

THINGS TO THINK ABOUT

1. What do I *love* to do?

2. What do I *think* I would like to learn, but I'm not sure?

3. What are my *dreams*? What do I need to do to chase those dreams?

DAY 4 Steps taken: _____   Miles journeyed: _____

Exercise chosen: _____

What I told God today: _____

_____

_____

_____

_____

Something I thought about: _____

_____

_____

_____

_____

Getting More Exercise

BIBLICAL BIG IDEA #5

*You must walk the precise path that the Lord your God indicates
for you so that you will live, and so that things will go well for
you, and so you will extend your time on the land that you will
possess.* —Deuteronomy 5:33

Exercise is good for you. God designed your body to move. You can
run, walk, bike, dance, do gymnastics, play basketball, play football, or
play soccer. You can play. Exercise is about moving your body and being
active; it is not supposed to be a chore. If you sit in front of a video game
or a TV all day, your body will waste away. When you do not move,
your muscles lose strength, your body gets weak, and your body stores
fat more readily. Humans are physical beings. Humans have relationships
with *real* people, not characters on TV or in games. Humans are meant
to move their bodies.

Video games and TV are fun and there is nothing wrong with doing
them for fun. However, video games and TV should not suck up all
your time. You need to balance play, games, sports, school, church, and
chores so you learn how to balance these things as an adult. The reason
that parents stress these activities now is because it is *much* easier to learn
new activities as a kid than as an adult. Your body is learning every day,
and when you learn these exercises now, your body will remember how
to continue to do these sports, exercises, and activities throughout your
entire life.

You have been wearing your fitness tracker for about five days now. Do
you like it? It is a good gauge to see how far you have moved in one day.
Adults need to move about 10,000 steps a day for health. Do you do that?
Can you beat that? Can you bike or walk to school? Can you run around
your neighborhood? Can you set a goal for how many laps up and down
your street you can run and then try to beat that over time? What games
can you play with your friends? Can you climb a tree? Can you go play in

a park? What do you think of signing up for your first race? Maybe your mom or dad would run it with you and train with you.

Getting exercise as a kid should be fun. Just go out there and be active. Enjoy the world God gave us.

THINGS TO THINK ABOUT

1. What do I like to do?

2. Is there a new exercise or sport that I would like to try?

3. How can I try something new?

4. How much time do I spend on TV and video games in a day?

5. Can I beat my mom or dad in their steps each day?

DAY 5 Steps taken: _____ Miles journeyed: _____

Exercise chosen: _____

What I told God today: _____

_____

_____

_____

_____

Something I thought about: _____

_____

_____

_____

_____

What Did God Make?

BIBLICAL BIG IDEA #6

Before I created you in the womb I knew you; before you were born I set you apart; I made you a prophet to the nations. —Jeremiah 1:5

God made many things. Most importantly, God made you. That makes you a very, very special person. I believe that God put each of us in the world for a purpose. I believe God put *you* here to do something special for the world, so let God work through you.

When we look at the world around us, we see many beautiful things. If you walk outside right now, count how many things you find beautiful. Do the colors, sounds, smells, sights, and tastes of the world around excite you? Do you wonder about this world? These are all things that we have because God created the world and the many people who have allowed God to work through them to make it a better place.

The Bible says we are stewards of God's world. That means we need to take care of the world we live in. Just as we show kindness to one another, we should show kindness to the earth and take care of the world in which we live.

God made you. God made the world, the earth, the solar system, and the universe. You are part of something much larger. What do you think about that?

THINGS TO THINK ABOUT

1. When I go outside, what are ten things I see, feel, hear, or taste that make me think of God?

2. What do I think about my role in the world around me?

3. How does it make me feel to be called special, important, and with a purpose?

DAY 6 Steps taken: _____ Miles journeyed: _____

Exercise chosen: _____

What I told God today: _____

_____

_____

_____

_____

Something I thought about: _____

_____

_____

_____

_____

7 Mama Told You to Eat Your Vegetables

BIBLICAL BIG IDEA #7

But on both banks of the river will grow up all kinds of fruit-bearing trees. Their leaves won't wither, and their fruitfulness won't wane. They will produce fruit in every month, because their water comes from the sanctuary. Their fruit will be for eating, their leaves for healing. —Ezekiel 47:12

In addition to you, God made the food we eat to make us strong and healthy to do God's work in the world. While your body is growing, it is important to put healthy food in it for fuel. Just like a sports car, your body is going to run better, move better, and perform better when you put a high-octane fuel in it. If you constantly fill your gas tank with chips, soda, cake, ice cream, and other junk, you are filling up your body with the wrong kind of "gas." Junk food is low-octane fuel for the machine that is your body.

If you want to go *fast*, be *strong*, and be full of *energy* in life, then you need to put high-performing gas in your "car" (your body). God did not hang "energy replacement food bars" on the trees in the Garden of Eden. God gave us fruits and vegetables, meats, fish, and fowl from which to choose. These are good foods and they are yummy foods. Experiment with the different tastes and flavors from the food God gave us and you will find that you will be more satisfied over time. Eating real food keeps your moods from going high and low and helps you feel less irritable. The chemicals and excess sugar in processed foods create signals in the brain almost like a drug—functioning like uppers and downers. Just like with any drug, your body has to come off of these chemicals that cause your moods to crash and burn. In moderation, your body is less likely to respond to this, but a steady diet of poor food choices leaves your body confused. It makes your body think it is on a non-stop roller coaster because it is not getting the food and nutrients it needs to function at a high level.

When you are irritable, you are more likely to make yourself, your parents, teachers, or siblings mad. So eating good foods is a good thing to do!

THINGS TO THINK ABOUT

1. What kind of food do I like to eat?

2. Is it food that God naturally gave me to eat?

3. Why do I like the food I like?

4. How does it make me feel to eat real food versus junk food?

5. Could I challenge myself to eat only food from God's earth for a day? A week? A month?

DAY 7 Steps taken: _____   Miles journeyed: _____

Exercise chosen: _____

What I told God today: _____

_____

_____

_____

_____

Something I thought about: _____

_____

_____

_____

_____

Don't Hit Your Sister (or Your Brother)

BIBLICAL BIG IDEA #8

You shall not take vengeance or bear a grudge against any of your people, but you shall love your neighbor as yourself I am the Lord. —Leviticus 19:18

Your brother or sister can be your best friend or your worst enemy. It is your choice how you get along with your sibling if you have one. God was clear when God said that we should first love one another.

Unfortunately, for you, this means you need to love your brother and/or sister. The commandment to love one another does not apply only outside of your family; it applies within it as well. Sometimes the hardest people to love are those that you have as relatives, but they can often be some of the strongest relationships you will ever have.

Consider this: Your sibling is the only person who will ever understand what it was like to be raised by your parent(s), or in the environment where you live. Your sibling has a shared experience of history that no one else will have. Sure, they may be annoying, but you have more things in common than you have differences if you think about it.

I am a little sister. Big brothers can be seriously annoying! However, this does not give me the right to hit, scream, yell mean things, or put shaving cream on my brother's pillow! Learning to get along with my brother taught me how to treat people right, even when I did not like them very much. If you look at the Bible stories, there are *many* incidents of siblings not getting along. It never ends well. God does not reward siblings that beat each other up, or worse, kill each other. Think about what happened to Cain and Abel! Rather, God rewards those siblings that have learned to forgive each other—think about Joseph and his coat of many colors with his brothers, or Jacob and Esau's relationship.

Moreover, your fights with your sibling makes your parent(s) nuts. God told us to honor our mother and father as well, and I am sure driving your parent(s) nuts does not count!

THINGS TO THINK ABOUT

1. Do I have a brother or sister? What do I think of my sibling?

2. What are three things my sibling and I have in common?

3. What are three things my sibling and I fight about?

4. What are three things my sibling and I can do to get along better?

DAY 8 Steps taken: _____ Miles journeyed: _____

Exercise chosen: _____

What I told God today: _____

_____

_____

_____

_____

Something I thought about: _____

_____

_____

_____

_____

9 Honor Your Body

BIBLICAL BIG IDEA #9

*They must teach my people the difference between the holy
and the ordinary, and show them the difference between clean
and unclean. —Ezekiel 44:23*

We have already established that God made you. God made *you* special
to do something *special* in the world. There is something the world needs
and you may be the best person to provide that to the world. God has
plans for you.

Paul tells us that our Christian calling is more than just having our
spirit directed to God. For example, your heart might be called to God,
but you can express your faith through your actions. We honor God
through what we do with our body: how we act, what we do, and how we
use it. God tells us that we are made in God's image and the Holy Spirit
is within us. On earth, the tool you have to do God's plan is your body.
This means your body is special too.

*Don't you know that your body is a temple of the Holy Spirit who is in you?
Don't you know that you have the Holy Spirit from God, and you don't
belong to yourselves? You have been bought and paid for, so honor God with
your body. —1 Corinthians 6:19–20*

What does this mean exactly? It means everything we do with our
bodies is for the glory of God. We should take care of our body because it
houses the Holy Spirit. What do you want to do with your body? Do you
want to get a tattoo? Do you want to get a piercing? Do you want to have
sex? Would you like to try drugs? Would you like to live on junk food?
I am not going to tell you what is right or wrong for you right now, but
when you think of the things you want to do, ask yourself, "What would
God do?" In addition, ask yourself, "What will I think about this in ten
years?" Does this decision honor God? If you are not sure, there is no

harm in waiting. Make your decisions through *thinking*, not just based on what you are feeling at any given moment.

If God is within me, and I have a reason for being here, then taking care of my body and honoring it is an important job. In fact, as we are growing up, taking care of the body is probably one of the most important things we can learn. You may think that what you do to your body now does not matter in the end, but all the decisions you are making now are shaping the life you will lead. We should not abuse our bodies. We should not abuse it with drugs, alcohol, promiscuous sex, cutting, junk food, tobacco, or other crap. Have a vision of yourself that you want to be and make your decisions each day based on meeting that goal.

THINGS TO THINK ABOUT

1. "God is in me." What do I think about that statement?

2. What are three things I do that are bad for my body?

3. What are three things I do that are good for my body?

4. What questions do I have about taking care of my body?

DAY 9   Steps taken: _____   Miles journeyed: _____

Exercise chosen: _____

What I told God today: _____

_____

_____

_____

_____

Something I thought about: _____

_____

_____

_____

_____

10 Make Good Choices

BIBLICAL BIG IDEA #10

But if it seems wrong in your opinion to serve the LORD, then choose today whom you will serve. Choose the gods whom your ancestors served beyond the Euphrates or the gods of the Amorites in whose land you live. But my family and I will serve the LORD. —Joshua 24:15

If there is one take away from this book that I want you to understand, it is this: *You* are responsible for *your* choices. Outside of the rules that your parent(s) are trying to teach you (and even then, it ends up being your choice if you learn to abide by rules), *you* make the choices about your life. *You* are responsible for *you*. No one else is responsible for your happiness but you and the choices you make.

Every choice has a consequence. Therefore, you need to think about the results of the choices you make and make sure that God is at the center of those choices. When you engage in a fight or an argument, you are making a choice. You always have the option to walk away or turn the other cheek. When you choose to drink, do drugs, or start smoking, *you* are making that choice. No one else is forcing you to do that. When you are growing up, the road less traveled is often the more difficult road because it requires that you learn to stand up for yourself and your beliefs. If you learn now to study the Bible and make decisions based on what Jesus taught, you often make the right choice. Now, there are times where the Bible has been used to do wrong, but that does not make the Bible wrong. If you look at the decisions made throughout history, ask yourself, did this decision honor God or show love to another?

When *you* make choices, ask yourself, "Does this honor God?" "Does this choice show love for others or me?" If your answer is "no," it is probably not the right decision.

Bad things happen in life. I cannot think of a single person I have met in my life who has not had some sort of tragedy hit them. Tragedy happens and bad things happen in life. They may have already happened to you. You can *choose* to blame these things for everything that is bad in your life, or the choices you make, or you can *choose* to rise above these events and still make good choices.

Again, no matter what happens to you, if you choose to love God and love others, you are probably making the right choice.

THINGS TO THINK ABOUT

1. What kind of tough choices do I have to make?

2. What is the right decision if I choose to love God and love others?

3. Have bad things happened to me? How did they make me feel? Do I think those bad things forced me to make choices, or did I choose to make the right choice in spite of them?

DAY 10 Steps taken: _____ Miles journeyed: _____

Exercise chosen: _____

What I told God today: _____

_____

_____

_____

_____

Something I thought about: _____

_____

_____

_____

_____

11 Talk to God

BIBLICAL BIG IDEA #11

*I say be guided by the Spirit and you won't carry out your
selfish desires.* —Galatians 5:16

When you cannot depend on anyone else, God will always be there. God *always* has an open ear even if you cannot feel, touch, or see God. We talk to God through prayer. Prayers come in many shapes, sizes, forms, and ways. Prayers do not have to be complex. Prayers can be a simple "God, I need you" or "God, thank you" or "God, help me." God understands far more about us than we understand about God, so do not think there is anything so complex in your life that God cannot help or understand. We build our relationship and understanding of God through prayer and study. When we study God's word (the Bible) and have a conversation with God (prayer), we begin to see and hear answers for our prayers.

There is nothing going on in your life that God cannot understand. Prayer allows us to share these thoughts, feelings, fears, anger, and frustrations in a constructive way. When we are silent after our prayers, we give ourselves the chance to hear God speak to us in our hearts. It is important to have the silent moments in prayer as well as the speaking moments so we give God a chance to answer. It is not only speaking to God that is a part of prayer, but also listening.

Prayer is a discipline. This means it is something you have to repeat every day for it to become a part of your life. Just like exercise, eating right, and learning to be kind, prayer requires that we practice it repeatedly for it to be a part of who we are and how we deal with life. Prayer lets us deal with life in a healthy manner. When I pray, I like to focus on my breathing while I say the words, or after when I am in listening mode. When you focus on your breath going in and out during prayer, it helps to slow your thoughts, heart rate, and blood pressure. Prayer provides a sense of calm in your body.

If you practice prayer as a habit, when you get frustrated you will find you are better able to tackle those things that bother you most. Practicing prayer also gives you a chance to think through the decisions you face. If you are not sure about what to do, pray about it before making a decision and then you will be more likely to make the right decision.

THINGS TO THINK ABOUT

1. As I practice a prayer, I will think about my breath while I pray and while I listen. What happened?

2. What sort of things would I like to ask God about, but are too afraid to ask?

3. What sort of things do I pray about?

DAY 11 Steps taken: _____ Miles journeyed: _____

Exercise chosen: _____

What I told God today: _____

_____

_____

_____

_____

Something I thought about: _____

_____

_____

_____

_____

The Difference between Right and Wrong

BIBLICAL BIG IDEA #12

The LORD proclaims: Do what is just and right; rescue the oppressed from the power of the oppressor. Don't exploit the refugee, the orphan, and the widow. Don't spill the blood of the innocent in this place. —Jeremiah 22:3

God did not send us out in the world without instructions on determining what is right and what is wrong. God gave us the Ten Commandments as a list of instructions so that we did not have to figure things out on our own. Humans have made multiple errors over time in determining right from wrong, and many have misinterpreted the Bible to justify what they were doing as right when in fact it was wrong. Slavery is a great example of how the Bible was misinterpreted. When humans have used the Bible for wrong versus right, it has come down to two things: Humans are fallible (this means we were born into sin and as a result, we often screw up) and we failed to follow God's top two commands:

He replied, "You must love the Lord your God with all your heart, with all your being, and with all your mind. This is the first and greatest commandment. And the second is like it: You must love your neighbor as you love yourself." —Matthew 22:37–39

When you are trying to determine right from wrong, ask yourself these two questions: Does this honor God? Does this show love for my neighbor (or friend, family, or person on the street)? "Neighbor" is considered a broad word in the Bible; it is anyone around you. If you cannot answer these questions in the affirmative, you should probably think about what you are doing, or go talk to someone you trust to help you make the right decision. There is no shame in asking for help. In fact, getting a second opinion on things from a trusted adult is often a smart choice. Even now as an adult, I really appreciate being able to reach out to a trusted friend to get opinions on the right thing to do when I have mixed feelings.

At the end of the day, when we make decisions based on love, we are doing the best job we can. I think God understands that. God appreciates love most of all, so when we make decisions based on love, we are doing our best.

THINGS TO THINK ABOUT

1. What are some hard decisions I have had to make?

2. How did I handle them?

3. Would my decisions have been any different if I had made those decisions based on God's Word and love?

DAY 12   Steps taken: _____   Miles journeyed: _____

Exercise chosen: _____

What I told God today: _____

_____

_____

_____

_____

Something I thought about: _____

_____

_____

_____

_____

13 It's Okay to Say That You Are Sorry

BIBLICAL BIG IDEA #13

I will heal their faithlessness; I will love them freely, for my anger has turned from them. —Hosea 14:4

It is difficult to love someone when we are angry with him or her. Perhaps they did something to you, or you did something to them, but a rift in the relationship has occurred and it can make it very difficult between you and that other person. This person may be a family member, a friend, someone you do not know well, or even a teacher or leader; but when that anger festers, it grows and grows in your heart.

Anger only gets smaller through forgiveness. It costs you *nothing* to forgive another person and grants you all the peace in the world. It costs you *nothing* but words to say "I am sorry," but gives you everything you need to move on. Forgiveness is like pouring water on the fire of your anger. Anger cannot thrive in an environment of forgiveness. When we forgive, our hearts are lighter, we are *happier*, and we are better able to continue with the work we are to do in the world.

Even at your age, you have a reason for being in this world. (I will tell you this over and over until you *believe* it.) For the most part, right now, your "job" is school and being a part of your family. You should take pride in doing those things well. When you have anger in your heart or an unresolved issue with another person, you do not do your job well. If you dwell on your anger and angst at this person, it begins to take over your mind, your attitude, and your life. School will suffer. Your relationships with your friends will suffer. Your relationship with your parents will suffer. Remember only you can control you. *You* have the ability to forgive and move on. That other person may not accept your forgiveness or even hear it, but *you* have taken control of your anger and made a step towards letting it go.

Forgiveness is freeing. God promised us that if we repent of our sins and ask for forgiveness for those things that we have done wrong, we will be forgiven. When we forgive or ask forgiveness, our sins are gone. God has promised this to us. We have the opportunity to do the same when we forgive others.

Above all, show sincere love to each other, because love brings about the forgiveness of many sins. —1 Peter 4:8

It is okay to say you are sorry. It costs you nothing.

THINGS TO THINK ABOUT

1. Is there someone I should forgive?

2. Is there something I need forgiveness for doing?

3. Do I feel uncomfortable saying I am sorry?

4. How do I feel when I'm forgiven?

DAY 13   Steps taken: _____   Miles journeyed: _____

Exercise chosen: _____

What I told God today: _____

_____

_____

_____

_____

Something I thought about: _____

_____

_____

_____

_____

14 What Is Lent, Anyway?

BIBLICAL BIG IDEA #14

He was in the wilderness forty days, tempted by Satan. He was among the wild animals, and the angels took care of him.
—Mark 1:13

Lent is a season during the church year that comes before Easter. Lent reminds us of the time in which Jesus went away from his disciples to go into the wilderness to fast (not eat or drink) for forty days and forty nights while focusing on prayer with God. Many people much smarter than me have debated exactly how Jesus survived for forty days and forty nights without food or drink. I do not need that level of specific understanding of what happened back then. I am comfortable with simply having faith.

When I read this passage, my understanding is that Jesus separated himself from the world for a long time, denying his human needs in order to focus on his spiritual needs and his relationship with God. During Lent, Christians (that includes me and you) are called to be more like Jesus during this time. This is one reason that Christ Walk makes a good Lenten discipline.

Different people have focused on becoming more like Jesus in many different ways. Some people give things up during Lent (sweets, bread, soda, arguing, whining, fighting) and other people take on new habits that they feel draw them closer to God (studying the Bible, working in a homeless shelter, doing a good deed each day, praying, walking, running, meditating). All of these habits make ourselves more like Jesus and thus closer to God. All of these are Christ Walk "miles" and activities.

In the Christ Walk program, we choose to walk steps and take on different activities that represent our relationship with God as a part of our journey. You may do this during Lent or during some other time of the year. *Anytime* is a good time to be more like Jesus. It does not only need to happen during Lent. At this point in your life, it is important for you to build habits that will instill discipline and bring you closer to God.

THINGS TO THINK ABOUT

1. What's a discipline?

2. What are some disciplines I can take on that bring me closer to God?

3. What are some habits that I need to give up in order to get closer to God?

4. How does it make me feel to give something up for a long period of time?

5. What do I think was on Jesus' mind when he was in the wilderness?

DAY 14   Steps taken: _____   Miles journeyed: _____

Exercise chosen: _____

What I told God today: _____

_____

_____

_____

_____

Something I thought about: _____

_____

_____

_____

_____

15 Why Did Jesus Die?

BIBLICAL BIG IDEA #15

God so loved the world that he gave his only Son, so that everyone who believes in him won't perish but will have eternal life. —John 3:16

Why did Jesus die? We are getting into some complicated ideas now. Bottom line: Jesus died for our sins, so that we would not have to make sacrifices to God in order to become reconciled to God. Jesus died to save us from *all* our sins. It was the ultimate gift of *love*. Jesus' death is love in action. Through his actions, we see that love will always win in every situation. God understood that we needed to see this very brutal end to realize that the only answer to any situation is to love one another first.

When God made a covenant with the Hebrews, they would originally make sacrifices of animals and gifts from the earth when they sinned (you can read Leviticus if you would like a *detailed* account of the types of sacrifices that could be made depending on the sin). These sacrifices were an outward sign of repentance for the sins that had been committed. People used sacrifices make things *right* with God (this is what we mean to be reconciled to God).

As time went on, God realized that there would need to be a really big sacrifice in order to reconcile the sinfulness of people with the righteousness of God. Jesus was this big sacrifice for us. Jesus loves us so much that he died for our sins. This love shows us that there is no greater gift than for each of us to love one another.

For the Human One didn't come to be served but rather to serve and to give his life to liberate many people. —Mark 10:45

Jesus died to show us *how* we should live for one another and how to love one another: selflessly. God realizes that we are flawed and we continue to sin, but the gift of Jesus' love, crucifixion, and resurrection give us hope that we can aspire to love as much as God loves us. The gift of Jesus' life gave *us* the promise of life everlasting with God if we follow in the way of Christ.

THINGS TO THINK ABOUT

1. Do my actions show the love of Jesus to those around me?

2. What can I do to be more like Christ each day?

3. What do I think it means to be saved by Jesus?

DAY 15 Steps taken: _____ Miles journeyed: _____

Exercise chosen: _____

What I told God today: _____

_____

_____

_____

_____

Something I thought about: _____

_____

_____

_____

_____

16 Why Did God Raise Jesus from the Dead?

BIBLICAL BIG IDEA #16

Christ died for our sins in line with the scriptures, he was buried, and he rose on the third day in line with the scriptures.
—1 Corinthians 15:3b–4

So . . . Jesus died for our sins. That is only part of the story. People die all the time. What was different about Jesus' death? It was brutal for sure. It was very painful. It was incredibly brave and sad and scary and unjust and all sorts of things. It was the right thing to do for the people of the world to have a future with God.

Then what happened? Jesus did not just die. He rose again on the third day. This is the miracle of the resurrection. Jesus came back to life after being dead for *three days*. This is a sign from God that God can overcome anything, even death, in order for us to have a relationship with God. God can make all things right. We have to *choose* to have a relationship with God in order for God to work through us to make things right in the world.

We are all a part of the resurrection miracle when we choose to honor and renew our Baptismal Covenant as being a part of the body of Christ. The church is the body of Christ in the world that continues the hope of resurrection for millions of people across the globe. You have a part in that big family of the church. We are a part of a miracle that changes lives every day when we choose to show love to one another. The gift of Jesus' resurrection shows us that there is promise in life. No matter how bad things have become, there is hope for a new beginning with God and a promise of peace and life everlasting. This is why God raised Jesus from the dead: To show us not to focus on worldly concerns, rather to focus on the promises of God.

THINGS TO THINK ABOUT

1. What do I think "life everlasting" means?

2. What do I think of miracles?

3. Does Jesus' death give me hope? How does it make me feel?

DAY 16   Steps taken: _____   Miles journeyed: _____

Exercise chosen: _____

What I told God today: _____

_____

_____

_____

_____

Something I thought about: _____

_____

_____

_____

_____

What Do I Do if I Make Mistakes?

BIBLICAL BIG IDEA #17

But if we confess our sins, he is faithful and just to forgive us our sins and cleanse us from everything we've done wrong.
—1 John 1:9

We all make mistakes. There is not a single person on earth that has not, or will not, make a mistake in life. Humans are inherently sinful and our struggle each day is to overcome our sinful desires and be more like Jesus. Although we try very hard not to sin, it is bound to happen.

Perhaps you said an unkind word. Perhaps you did an unkind deed. Perhaps you lied. Perhaps you argued with your parent(s), or hit your brother or sister. Perhaps you stole, or broke a law. Perhaps you have done something you think is unforgiveable. You are wrong. God has promised us that if we confess our sins and present a contrite heart for what we have done, we have forgiveness. Now, you cannot ask forgiveness and go right back to doing what you did that was wrong. Part of confessing sins is trying not to repeat them in the future. When you present a contrite heart to God, you are giving your best effort to walk in Jesus' steps and not make those same mistakes again.

God is very forgiving. God understands all our desires, our fears, and the things we do wrong. When we confess our sins and try to make things right after mistakes, we feel better. The act of contrition and forgiveness heals our hearts and makes it possible for us to go on in the world trying to do the work of God around us.

If you are not sure how to ask for forgiveness, God knows better than we do what we have done wrong. There are prayers we can pray that outline our transgressions as humans and provide us words to articulate to God our desire to do a better job:

THE GENERAL CONFESSION
Most merciful God,
    we confess that we have sinned against you
    in thought, word, and deed,
by what we have done,
and what we have left undone.
We have not loved you with our whole heart;
we have not loved our neighbors as ourselves.
We are truly sorry and we humbly repent.
for the sake of your Son Jesus Christ,
have mercy on us and forgive us;
that we may delight in your will,
and walk in your ways,
to the glory of your Name. Amen.
    —The Book of Common Prayer, 1979, p. 360

THINGS TO THINK ABOUT

1. Do I have something that weighs on my heart and needs forgiveness?

2. What parts of the General Confession stand out to me?

3. What do I think about forgiveness?

DAY 17 Steps taken: _____ Miles journeyed: _____

Exercise chosen: _____

What I told God today: _____

_____

_____

_____

_____

Something I thought about: _____

_____

_____

_____

_____

18 Will God Always Love Me?

BIBLICAL BIG IDEA #18

I am convinced that nothing can separate us from God's love in Christ Jesus our Lord: not death or life, not angels or rulers, not present things or future things, not powers or height or depth, or any other thing that is created. —Romans 8:38–39

Just like the song we learned when we were little: *Jesus loves me, this I know*, these words continue to ring with truth. Many times, as we grow older and we do stupid things, we begin to think that we have done so many bad things that God cannot possibly continue to forgive us and love us anyway.

One of the great mysteries of our faith is that God continues to be faithful. The Bible is a documentation of God's faith to God's people over centuries of sin and wrongdoing. God continues to forgive God's people and the people that God loves. There are people in this world that have done much more wrong than you, but God continues to forgive and provide a path for redemption. This means that somewhere in the middle of evilness, God can prevail.

When you feel unloved, pray. Connect with God, because God loves you more than anything. Remember, you were created for a reason and that reason was love. No matter what you do in life and no matter where you go and no matter how far you may stray from the path, God will always, always, always love you.

THINGS TO THINK ABOUT

1. Do I really think it's possible that God can love me no matter what?

2. Do I think I am loveable?

3. What ways do I think that God shows us that God loves us?

DAY 18 Steps taken: _____ Miles journeyed: _____

Exercise chosen: _____

What I told God today: _____

_____

_____

_____

_____

Something I thought about: _____

_____

_____

_____

_____

19 Your Body Is a Temple

BIBLICAL BIG IDEA #19

*When you walk, you won't be hindered; when you run,
you won't stumble. —Proverbs 4:12*

On Day 9, we talked about how to "Honor Your Body." This chapter is a
continuation of that, because I think it is important for you to understand
that your body is a temple of the Holy Spirit on Earth.

*Do you not know that your body is a temple of the Holy Spirit who is in you?
Don't you know that you have the Holy Spirit from God, and you don't belong
to yourselves? You have been bought and paid for, so glorify God with your body.
—1 Corinthians 6:19–20*

Your body is important. It is your job to take care of it. Do not abuse
your body. We tend to take out our frustrations in life on our bodies.
Right now, you are creating habits that will build a strong and healthy
temple for a long and healthy life. As we get older, we tend to substitute
healthy habits with unhealthy ones. For example, your boyfriend or girl-
friend broke up with you, so you decide to eat a gallon of ice cream, or
start smoking, or worse yet, hurt yourself or someone else. None of these
decisions starts from a position of love.

When we are growing up (and this often applies to adults as well),
we tend to *react* to situations. The smartest lesson you can learn is *not* to
react with your first impulse. Take a moment to think through what you
are feeling and what you want to do. Consider the consequences of the
decisions you make. Some decisions in life cannot be changed once you
make them. If you hurt someone or yourself, you have made a decision
for a lifetime that has ramifications far beyond just you. If you decide to
go out and get a tattoo or a piercing, then you are stuck with that for the
rest of your life. If that is what you want, then that is fine; I am just telling
you to think it through before reacting.

If you learn to respond to stresses to your body by feeding it junk food, or drugs, or alcohol, then you are making decisions that affect it for the rest of your life. You are not treating your body like a temple of God when you make these kinds of decisions when you are *reacting*.

Rather, take this approach in a situation: Stop. Breathe. Pray.

Ask yourself does this decision *love God*? Does this decision *love me*? Does this decision *love someone else*?

If you cannot answer the affirmative to those questions, you might want to think of alternatives to your decision. Otherwise, you may be faced with the consequences for the rest of your life.

THINGS TO THINK ABOUT

1. What are some tough choices I have to make about my body?

2. Have there been consequences? Are there consequences?

3. What do I think about the consequences of the decisions I've made so far? Am I okay with them?

DAY 19 Steps taken: _____ Miles journeyed: _____

Exercise chosen: _____

What I told God today: _____

_____

_____

_____

Something I thought about: _____

_____

_____

_____

_____

20 Why Do We Get Sick?

BIBLICAL BIG IDEA #20

Have mercy on me, O LORD, because I'm frail. Heal me, LORD, because my bones are shaking in terror! —Psalm 6:2

Illness happens. Just like our souls, our bodies are also flawed. Disease, sickness, and disability occur because our bodies are imperfect. Our bodies react to things in the world and environmental changes to which we are exposed. Our bodies react to new germs and new parasites in known and unknown ways. Our bodies react to the food, drugs, and chemicals we put in it that may have long-term effects that we do not initially see.

There are many reasons we get sick. Not all of them make a whole lot of sense. I live a healthy life of exercise, good diet, and prayer. I still got cancer. My genetic make-up is such that my immune system does not fight the cancer cells well. My illness is just one of those things that happen. It could have been environmental toxins that I was exposed to that changed my system. It may have been something that happened because of a virus. There are many different thoughts on why different kinds of illnesses occur and why they happen to some people and not to other people.

Many habits help our bodies fight off sickness and disease. Eat a well-balanced diet with lots of real food including fruits and vegetables, get plenty of exercise and sleep, wash your hands, pray, and play. Will this ensure you *never* get sick? No, not at all. I am a good example that things sometimes just happen. However, it will keep you healthier and stronger to deal with whatever may happen to your body.

There are different levels of illness. Some are everyday illnesses—not all sicknesses are a bad thing. Sometimes we get sick so that our bodies learn how to fight foreign germs in the body. This is a good thing as it builds your immune system. Nevertheless, illnesses that are more serious threaten our life and wellbeing. It is important that as you are growing you build those habits in your life that help protect you from those serious illnesses, or make you stronger to live with them in your daily life.

THINGS TO THINK ABOUT

1. Do I have a serious illness? How do my daily habits help me stay strong?

2. What are my healthy habits?

3. How do I feel about being sick?

DAY 20   Steps taken: _____   Miles journeyed: _____

Exercise chosen: _____

What I told God today: _____

_____

_____

_____

_____

Something I thought about: _____

_____

_____

_____

_____

21 Take Care of the Earth

BIBLICAL BIG IDEA #21

For this is what the LORD said, who created the heavens, who is God, who formed the earth and made it, who established it, who didn't create it a wasteland but formed it as a habitation: I the LORD, and none other! —Isaiah 45:18

God gave people dominion over the earth. This is not lordship over the world. This is not a suppressive approach to care of the world. Rather, it is a duty and a responsibility of humans to take care of this world that God gave us for our home.

Our world is a living, breathing entity. The choices we make in this world affect the earth we live on. We might not see the impact of our choices on the earth immediately. Often, things that we do on earth have consequences many years down the line. Remember that the choices you make today have an impact for generations to come.

It is hard to think like this. The key to remember is that your choices are not made in a bubble. When you spit your gum on the sidewalk, it has consequences: it could stick to someone's shoe, an animal could try to eat it and choke, or it could be poisonous to a bird and kill it. When you litter, you contribute to a dirty world that attracts disease-laden rodents, you leave trash that makes for an ugly environment, and you end up not putting things were they could be recycled. If that trash goes into a lake or other body of water, it creates pollution that creates an imbalance in the chemistry of that water that goes on to impact the life of many creatures that live and thrive in that water.

It is our responsibility to take care of the earth. Think about what you are doing. Does your decision love the earth and all the animals within it? The fish, fowl, and animals in this world are our neighbors, too. Let us take care of them.

THINGS TO THINK ABOUT

1. How do I take care of God's earth?

2. What are some things we can all do to help take care of the earth better?

3. What are some decisions of the past that we are living with today in the world?

DAY 21   Steps taken: _____   Miles journeyed: _____

Exercise chosen: _____

What I told God today: _____

_____

_____

_____

_____

Something I thought about: _____

_____

_____

_____

_____

22 Take Care of Your Friends

BIBLICAL BIG IDEA #22

He denounces his friends for gain, and his children's eyes fail.
—Job 17:5

We are supposed to love our neighbors as ourselves. Our friends are our neighbors. Our friends, especially ones we click with for a lifetime, will be those that hold us up through the storms of life. My friends are my "posse." They are the people I talk to when I am not sure what my problems are and to see how they have handled similar situations. My friends have my back. We jokingly call this, "We are Groot." Groot, from *Guardians of the Galaxy*, takes care of his friends. Groot wraps his friends in his deep roots to protect them from danger. Groot also comes back to life because his roots are strong and his relationships with his friends go deep. Groot has his friends' backs. Together, the Guardians are far stronger than if they were acting apart.

To have good friends, you first need to be a good friend. Good friends build you up. They do not tear you down. Similarly, you should build your friends up. Help them make good decisions, just as you are learning to make good decisions. Be each other's Groot. Groot is strong because his roots grow deep. Your friendship will grow strong as your roots grow deep with each other. Friends can last a lifetime if they are the right friends. They are the sorts of people that you can pick up a conversation with after ten years, and it is as though the initial conversation never ended. Lifetime friends are those whose love continues to grow no matter how far apart they may be. Lifetime friends are God's gift to us. Your friends should not lead you down a path of self-destruction. If your "friends" are urging you to do things that do not show love to yourself, the people around you, or your parents, they are not real friends. Friends love one another.

Taking care of our friends shows the covenant of God's love for us with one another. It shows love to ourselves, to one another, and to the world around us. Having good friends and being a good friend teaches us the discipline of how we should treat other people. Good friends show forgiveness, kindness, support, love, and caring. These are all things we should be cultivating not only for our friends and family but also for everyone around us.

THINGS TO THINK ABOUT

1. How am I a good friend?

2. Do I have a good friend?

3. What do I think makes my friendships special?

4. Do I talk with my friends about God? Would I like to?

DAY 22 Steps taken: _____ Miles journeyed: _____

Exercise chosen: _____

What I told God today: _____

_____

_____

_____

_____

Something I thought about: _____

_____

_____

_____

_____

Turning the Other Cheek

BIBLICAL BIG IDEA #23

You have heard that it was said, An eye for an eye and a tooth for a tooth. But I say to you that you must not oppose those who want to hurt you. If people slap you on your right cheek, you must turn the left cheek to them as well. When they wish to haul you to court and take your shirt, let them have your cloak too. —Matthew 5:38–40

When people do something wrong to us, our immediate reaction is to retaliate. We want vengeance, justice, and payback. We want to feel validated for our feelings. The problem is that Jesus calls us to turn the other cheek.

Common interpretation of "turning the other cheek" tells us that when a person hits you on one cheek, you should turn the other cheek and let that person hit you on the other cheek as well. This would lead us to assume that Jesus is advocating for tolerating abuse. On the contrary, Jesus would not tolerate abuse because it does not stem from a position of love. However, when Jesus does tell us to turn the other cheek, what he is trying to teach us is that retaliating with violence or aggression is not going to solve the problem that is occurring. You can stand up for yourself, your beliefs, and others without resorting to brutality. Does hitting your siblings back ever solve the immediate problem of your disagreement?

Remember, Jesus is trying to teach us to react from a position of love as our initial response to any situation. If I start from a position of love, then I would turn the other cheek. If I respond from a position of love, then my response will be to try to find out what is causing this act of aggression. If I respond from a position of love, then my goal will be to resolve the problem without violence. If I respond from a position of love, I will try to help this person. There is only one type of situation in which violence may be an okay response, and even then, you need to think carefully about your choice. Aggression in order to protect yourself, another person, or a group of people from harm may be the only response in a small number of situations. The key here is those are the exceptions, not the norm. In our everyday life, we are called to respond from a place of love. Violence is not from a place of love. Jesus is calling us to turn the other cheek so that we learn not react to every situation. As my daddy used to tell me, "Anna, soft overcomes hard." Eventually, love will win out if we all learn to respond from a place of love instead of violence.

THINGS TO THINK ABOUT

1. Is it hard to turn the other cheek?

2. What are some times when I have or have not turned the other cheek?

3. What are some examples of how to respond from a place of love in a charged situation?

DAY 23   Steps taken: _____   Miles journeyed: _____

Exercise chosen: _____

What I told God today: _____

_____

_____

_____

_____

Something I thought about: _____

_____

_____

_____

_____

Why Should I Pray?

BIBLICAL BIG IDEA #24

*L*ORD *my God, listen to your servant's prayer and request, and hear the cry and prayer that your servant prays to you today.*
—1 Kings 8:28

Prayer is our opportunity to develop a relationship with God. When you do not communicate, it is very difficult to build a relationship with anyone, let alone God. Prayer is the chance to talk to God. It gets the stuff that we all carry on our hearts out of our systems and in the hands of a loving God who can carry our worries, concerns, and wishes for us when they are too much for us to handle on our own. When we pray, it allows us to organize our thoughts and feelings about issues. When we pray, and then follow with silence, we give God the opportunity to weigh in on our thoughts, concerns, and issues in order to provide guidance to us in our daily lives. When we pray for others, our collective prayers wrap our friends and family in love so they are not alone on their journey.

Prayer is another physical discipline that teaches us to think, talk, and pray about our lives before we act upon them. Think about the results of things that you have done in the past. Would the outcome of any of your actions be different if you had prayed about it first?

What if your best friend says something to you that hurts your feelings? What if you say something equally mean back to him or her? Perhaps now, you are not speaking to each other. What if you had prayed about this first? Would the outcome have been different?

What if you were offered drugs or alcohol at a party? What if you prayed about that first? Would you have taken the drugs or alcohol? Would it have made you pause if you thought about what God would say to do?

Prayer is a pause button. Prayer provides us the opportunity to stop and think about what we are doing in all aspects of our lives. One of our greatest sins as humans is our propensity to *react* first without thinking through on our actions and praying about what God would want us to do.

THINGS TO THINK ABOUT

1. What are some things that I think would be a good idea to pray about first?

2. Are there times in my life when I wish I had prayed about something before reacting?

3. Are there situations in which prayer has helped me make a better decision?

DAY 24   Steps taken: _____   Miles journeyed: _____

Exercise chosen: _____

What I told God today: _____

_____

_____

_____

_____

Something I thought about: _____

_____

_____

_____

_____

25 How to Pray

BIBLICAL BIG IDEA #25

In the same way, the Spirit comes to help our weakness. We don't know what we should pray, but the Spirit himself pleads our case with unexpressed groans. —Romans 8:26

When we do not know what to pray or when we are not sure of the words to use, God has given us the Lord's Prayer in which to offer our prayers and supplications. You cannot go wrong when praying the words of the Lord's Prayer.

When you want to take your prayer to a different level, you need to pray from your heart. There are no wrong words in a dialogue with God. Honesty and forthrightness about your cares, concerns, sins, and worries are such things to pray to God.

Lord, my God, listen to your servant's prayer and request, and hear the cry and prayer that I your servant pray to you. —2 Chronicles 6:19

We should pray for forgiveness for what we have done wrong. It is a good discipline to name and understand those things we have done wrong, or not done, and to understand *why* they are wrong. We should pray for others. God hears many prayers. God hears each one of our petitions. We should lift each other up in prayer and pray for people by name and by need for healing, grace, forgiveness, loneliness, and reconciliation.

We should pray for reconciliation. We want to be right with God. We want to ensure that our path is following the path that God has set out for ourselves, not the one we set. We should pray to be reconciled with others when we are not getting along with friends, family, and colleagues.

We should give prayers of thanksgiving. God has blessed far more than we can hope to imagine. It is important to remember all those blessings and give thanks for them. When we remember what we have, the things we do not have seem smaller.

We can use prayers that others have written, we can pray our catechism (our set of beliefs from the church that begins on page 845 of the Episcopal Book of Common Prayer), and we can pray words from the Bible. But we can also just open our hearts and minds to God. We can have a conversation with God about all that is and all that will be in our lives.

We should pray every day. We will not develop the discipline of prayer if we do not practice it ourselves. I will pray for you, if you pray for me.

THINGS TO THINK ABOUT

1. Do I pray? Every day?

2. What do I pray about?

3. What do I struggle to pray about?

DAY 25 Steps taken: _____ Miles journeyed: _____

Exercise chosen: _____

What I told God today: _____

_____

_____

_____

_____

Something I thought about: _____

_____

_____

_____

_____

26 Talking to Someone We Can't See or Hear

BIBLICAL BIG IDEA #26

Therefore, go and make disciples of all nations, baptizing them in the name of the Father and of the Son and of the Holy Spirit, teaching them to obey everything that I've commanded you. Look, I myself will be with you every day until the end of this present age.—Matthew 28:19–20

Who is God? What does God look like? How can God really hear prayers when I cannot see, hear, or know that someone "real" is there? I do not really have any good answers for this. One of the ways we know God's presence is the feeling we have in our hearts when we practice the discipline of prayer. It is also seeing the hand of God in all things around us. Part of it is the understanding that the elegance and symmetry of the universe could only be made by God. There are signs of God all around us, in us, and in the love of others to each other. God is simply *everywhere*.

It may feel weird at first talking to someone you cannot see or hear like you would talk to your mom or dad, but God is there. It is something I am *very* sure about. Just as with anything a little weird at first, you have to repeat the discipline repeatedly for it to become comfortable and a part of who you are and how you live your life.

Think back to when you were learning to tie your shoes. That felt *weird*. It looked weird, and you had to get both of your hands working in concert with those slippery shoelaces. Then you had to do it repetitively before it became second nature.

Talking to God is like that. It feels really weird and uncomfortable at first, but if you do it time after time, it feels more right than wrong.

THINGS TO THINK ABOUT

1. Every day we have faith in things we do not see or hear: why would God be different?

2. Why does it feel weird to have a conversation with someone who isn't there?

3. Do I think I have a discipline of prayer in my life? How does it feel?

DAY 26   Steps taken: _____   Miles journeyed: _____

Exercise chosen: _____

What I told God today: _____

_____

_____

_____

_____

Something I thought about: _____

_____

_____

_____

_____

27 What If Mom or Dad Goes Away?

BIBLICAL BIG IDEA #27

Have mercy on me, Lord! Just look how I suffer because of those who hate me. But you are the one who brings me back from the very gates of death. —Psalm 9:13

Some kids do not have two parents. Some kids have more than two parents. Some kids start with two parents and then lose them. Some kids do not know their parents. Other kids have adoptive parents. Kids come with parents in all sorts of shapes, sizes, colors, identities, and creeds.

I like to think that *most* parents try really hard doing the best they can with the skills they have to raise their children. I know I *pray* very hard that I am doing the right job raising my kids. I love my kids so very much. I hope you know that those who care for you love you very much too. However, things can happen to parents too. Parents struggle with illness, tragedy, death, stress, and choices just as you do. Life and tragedy happen to all of us at some point in our lives. Parents would like to protect their kids from anything bad happening, but bad stuff happens all the time. Bad things will happen, but I think we need to learn how to live joyfully *in spite* of these things.

I was recently diagnosed with cancer. That means our family talked a lot about what would happen if I died. It was a very scary conversation for both my kids and me. Maybe you have been in that situation too. It is incredibly scary to think of your mom or dad going away. Especially when there is a lot of love wrapped up in your relationships. There are a couple of thoughts I have on this subject since it has hit close to home recently:

- *God* is not taking your parent away. *God* did not give me cancer. These things just happen in life. God is here with my family and me through anything that might happen. God will be there with *you* if you let God be a part of your life.

- You are tougher than you look. Kids are resilient. In the face of adversity, you will find a way to hold tight to precious memories and make new ones with the life you have.

- Your other parent or caregiver will be there—knit yourselves tightly together in love.

- Pray. Pray until the hurt goes away. Pray fiercely for God to help you through whatever you are going through. Pray for your parents, your siblings, and yourself. When nothing makes sense in life, prayer is often the only answer. Pray until you turn blue in the face. Pray and pray and pray.

Things that happen in life may not make sense, but you will find that no matter what happens to you or your parents, God has this amazing ability to take something awful and turn it into something beautiful.

THINGS TO THINK ABOUT

1. Have I had to think about losing a parent?

2. How did that make me feel?

3. What scares me the most about it? What are some ways I can find beauty in even the most awful of things?

DAY 27   Steps taken: _____   Miles journeyed: _____

Exercise chosen: _____

What I told God today: _____

_____

_____

_____

_____

Something I thought about: _____

_____

_____

_____

_____

Honor Your Mother and Your Father

BIBLICAL BIG IDEA #28

Honor your father and your mother so that your life will be long on the fertile land that the LORD your God is giving you.
—Exodus 20:12

You did not come with an instruction manual. It is the hardest thing in the world for a parent to teach you discipline, character, how to build a relationship with God, limits, and still show you all how much you are loved. I personally try to parent from a place of love, but it does not always come out that way. Parenting is tough. I am sure you have thought your parents were unfair, unkind, did not love you, and all sorts of things like that. I am sure I thought those things about my own parents when I was growing up too.

At the end of the day, though, God has commanded us to honor our mother and our father. Unless you are being abused or are in danger in your home life, parents are trying to teach you how to be a productive and responsible member of society when you grow up. If you are suffering from abuse, there is no excuse for this. It is not your fault—get help. For everyone else, try not to fight with your parents too much.

I think it is *very* important to recognize that in God's Ten Commandments, one of them is specifically about our relationship with our mother and our father. You do not have to agree with your mom or dad, but you do have to honor the fact that they are trying to teach you how to live from a perspective of how they grew up themselves. I can guarantee you that you will not agree with how your parents are trying to raise you. You will not agree with their style, their methods, or their approaches. There will be things you think they do correctly, and there will be many things that you think they did wrong. I can guarantee that when *you* have kids, *your* kids will think the same thing about you. There is no such thing as perfect parenting. Even the things you think you are doing absolutely right could be wrong for the child you have. Parenting is a constant learning experience. *Most* parents are just trying to do the best job they can, so keep that in mind when you do not agree with them.

I can tell you from experience that they will be far more inclined to listen to you if you talk to them reasonably. They might not change their minds, but if you talk to them (and not scream, yell, and stamp your feet), this will go a long way to honoring your parents. Have a conversation rather than a fight about the topic you want to discuss. Remember—parents are trying to parent from a place of love. Your response to them should be from a place of love as well.

THINGS TO THINK ABOUT

1. How is my relationship with my parent(s)?

2. What things do I think my parents do right?

3. What things do I think my parents do wrong?

4. How can I approach my communication with them to improve on those things that bother me?

DAY 28   Steps taken: _____   Miles journeyed: _____

Exercise chosen: _____

What I told God today: _____

_____

_____

_____

_____

Something I thought about: _____

_____

_____

_____

_____

29 Don't Steal

BIBLICAL BIG IDEA #29
Do not steal. —Exodus 20:15

Another commandment from God is not to steal. You have your stuff; other people have their stuff. Not all people have equal stuff. Stealing things that do not belong to you is not right. Do not do it.

When you steal, you may have taken something of value from one person. Perhaps you are stealing items from a store that provides the livelihood of the owner of that store. There are effects of stealing on the person you are stealing from, the people that work for them, and their families.

Stealing has an impact on you and your family. If you are caught (and eventually you will be), you will get in trouble. Your parents may have to pay for what you have stolen. *You* should have to pay for what you have stolen. You could go to jail if the infraction is severe enough. This could influence your schooling, your future jobs, and what responsibilities people trust you with in the future.

Stealing is just flat out wrong. It does not come from a place of love. There is not a good solid reason to steal. The thrill of "getting away with it" is not worth it in the end. Do not do it. Do not let your friends do it, and do not let them talk you into it.

THINGS TO THINK ABOUT

1. Have I ever stolen anything? Have I ever thought about stealing?

2. Why?

3. How can I take responsibility for those actions?

DAY 29 Steps taken: _____   Miles journeyed: _____

Exercise chosen: _____

What I told God today: _____

_____

_____

_____

_____

Something I thought about: _____

_____

_____

_____

_____

DAY •
30 Do Not Desire Stuff

BIBLICAL BIG IDEA #30

Do not desire your neighbor's house. Do not desire and try to take your neighbor's wife, male or female servant, ox, donkey, or anything that belongs to your neighbor. —Exodus 20:17

I am a big fan of reduce, reuse, and recycle. I grew up with a grandfather who would fix or reuse just about everything rather than buying anything new. In the grand scheme of things, stuff is just stuff. You will not take your stuff to heaven. You really do not need stuff so do not worry about your stuff.

Your accumulated stuff ends up being garbage the world has to do something with when you throw it away. We should try to minimize the amount of stuff we just discard. Can we do something else with it? Is there someone else who may need it more? Do we really need more stuff to replace the stuff we have?

As you grow up, having stuff seems incredibly important. We want the coolest clothes, hippest electronics, and neatest toys. Stuff is just material goods. Stuff is not as important as it may seem. It is not. Value what you have, don't desire more than that, or what your friends have, and think really hard about adding more stuff to your stash. When we focus so much on the things we want and think we "need" we often forget those who are without. Couldn't we spend our money on things that *other* people really need to live? Do we really need to add more stuff to our own pockets?

Think about what stuff you really *need*. Then, focus on helping others get the stuff they need to survive. Some stuff really helps us take care of our neighbors. Other stuff just adds junk to our lives that we do not need. Remember, you can't take your stuff with you in the next life. Will you really want or care about this needless stuff anymore?

59

THINGS TO THINK ABOUT

1. What do I think about stuff?

2. Do I have a lot of stuff? Do I feel like I need more stuff?

3. What is the difference between a want and a need?

DAY 30   Steps taken: _____   Miles journeyed: _____

Exercise chosen: _____

What I told God today: _____

_____

_____

_____

_____

Something I thought about: _____

_____

_____

_____

_____

Waiting for Love

BIBLICAL BIG IDEA #31

[Man] Look at you—so beautiful, my dearest! Look at you—
so beautiful! Your eyes are doves! [Woman] Look at you—so
beautiful, my love! Yes, delightful! Yes, our bed is lush and
green! —Song of Solomon 1:15–16

As you get older, your body will change and grow. All the hormones in your body, no matter your age, send signals to your brain signaling hunger, want, need, love, pain, anxiety, and many other feelings. As you grow up, it is important to become aware of the signals your body sends and respond to them with your brain, not just your heart and feelings. One of the things that you will struggle with as you grow up are the signals that your body sends you about other people. Especially when you feel very strongly that you like or love someone. The initial feelings of love and attraction are *very* strong, especially when you are young. It is a wonderful, exciting feeling to be attracted to someone, but those feelings can often take over making good decisions.

If you are not sure about sex, or having sex with someone, there is *zero* harm in waiting. In fact, sex and the consequences of sex (pregnancy, sexually transmitted diseases, commitments, marriage, and more) are significant. I think you should wait to have sex until marriage because it is complicated. God intended for us to have sexual relations with someone that we are committed to for *life*.

My daddy told me (or rather he told my brother and I was listening in on the conversation), "We think you should wait to have sex for marriage, but if you don't, you better be protected." If you have sex outside of marriage, there are consequences: things like pregnancy and disease that could affect you for the rest of your life. You need to think about the consequences of having sex at any age. Sex is not just about how good it may feel and how awesome it may be to love someone. Sex is far more complicated that an act of coming together with someone.

Sex has consequences. There is *zero* error in waiting to have sex until you are absolutely sure in your heart *and* mind that it is the right thing to do.

THINGS TO THINK ABOUT

1. Is it okay to wait to have sex until I am married? (Really, it is okay to wait.) Do I have to prove I love someone by having sex with him or her before marriage?

2. What do I think about sex?

3. Do I think sex is part of a commitment to a lifelong relationship?

4. What do I think God says about sex?

DAY 31 Steps taken: _____   Miles journeyed: _____

Exercise chosen: _____

What I told God today: _____

_____

_____

_____

_____

Something I thought about: _____

_____

_____

_____

_____

What Is a Covenant?

BIBLICAL BIG IDEA #32

I am now setting up my covenant with you, with your descendants. —Genesis 9:9

A covenant is a binding agreement between two people, or between God and God's people. God made a covenant with the people of Israel that God would take care of them if they were God's people. Marriage is a covenant between two people who have committed to loving each other and living life together. A Baptismal Covenant is made between you and God (and your parents and godparents) during your baptism that marks you as Christ's own forever. When you are confirmed (if you choose to do so), you acknowledge and bind yourself to your Baptismal Covenant as an adult.

Covenants are holy agreements. They are your word and your heart invested in a relationship with God or another person. Covenants should not be broken. They are "for-life" agreements. Does that make the agreement easy to keep? Not at all—life happens that makes these agreements difficult to keep. When I got my cancer, I really felt that God had broken a covenant with me. It was not true, but I was so hurt by what my body had done to betray me that the only thing that could handle the anger I felt was God. God kept his covenant and continues to love and take care of me despite my cancer. He has healed me from the pain of my disease, although I am not cured. This is a mighty distinction. You can still have troubles, but the covenant can remain intact as you work through the issues.

In the case of covenants between people, there are things that can break those covenants: adultery (cheating on someone), abuse, breaking your word. Remember, entering into a covenant is an important, special, and holy thing. God has a special covenant with you. God will never leave you and never stop loving you, no matter what happens in your life. Even when you feel the furthest from God, God will always honor your covenant.

Covenants are holy. Treat them as such.

THINGS TO THINK ABOUT

1. What do I think about covenants?

2. Do I have a covenant with God or someone right now?

3. Do I think it is okay to break covenants?

DAY 32 Steps taken: _____ Miles journeyed: _____

Exercise chosen: _____

What I told God today: _____

_____

_____

_____

_____

Something I thought about: _____

_____

_____

_____

_____

How Far Do I Have to Walk to Be Healthy?

BIBLICAL BIG IDEA #33

So then let's run the race that is laid out in front of us, since we have such a great cloud of witnesses surrounding us. Let's throw off any baggage, get rid of the sin that trips us up, and fix our eyes on Jesus, faith's pioneer and perfecter. He endured the cross, ignoring the shame, for the sake of the joy that was laid out in front of him, and sat down at the right side of God's throne. —Hebrews 12:1–3

Taking care of your body is a lifelong effort. As we have discussed for the last thirty-plus days, it includes all sorts of mind, body, and spiritual disciplines that make you healthy. Healthy does not just mean exercise; healthy includes all the actions that keep your heart, mind, body, and soul whole.

You will work on these disciplines your entire life. It does not end. Right now as you are growing, your goal is to establish those behaviors that make for a healthy body now. It is *much* harder to learn when you are older.

Science tells us that we need to be active for thirty minutes or longer on most days of the week. These numbers change all the time, but it is a good guideline for setting goals. You can also set goals to move at least 10,000 steps a day as that is another benchmark that the experts use. Getting up for five minutes for every hour of sitting keeps you moving. Trying to eat fruits and vegetables with every meal ensures you get a mix of the right vitamins and nutrients to keep you healthy. Taking three, fifteen-minute walks throughout the day will keep you moving. Playing a sport, playing with friends, biking, hiking, swimming, or whatever activity floats your boat, will keep you active for a lifetime.

There is no magic bullet that will protect you from disease. However, there are minimum standards that help keep your body healthy. The bottom line is you need to be active and keep moving. That is what will keep you healthy. When we quit moving and stop being active, the body gets sluggish and stops performing like a well-oiled machine. Just as your parents take care of their cars with maintenance, check-ups, and diagnostics, you need to do the same thing for your body throughout your life.

Keep walking. Keep moving and keep making decisions that help to keep you healthy for the long term.

THINGS TO THINK ABOUT

1. Am I moving enough?

2. Have I increased my activity through this program?

3. How am I making choices that will build a healthy body for a long life?

4. If I am not, what else should I think about doing?

DAY 33   Steps taken: _____   Miles journeyed: _____

Exercise chosen: _____

What I told God today: _____

_____

_____

_____

_____

Something I thought about: _____

_____

_____

_____

_____

DAY 34 Asking for Forgiveness

BIBLICAL BIG IDEA #34

Know now then that the LORD your God is the only true God! He is the faithful God, who keeps the covenant and proves loyal to everyone who loves him and keeps his commands—even to the thousandth generation! —Deuteronomy 7:9

Big News Bulletin: God is *very* forgiving. God has forgiven prostitutes, alcoholics, drug addicts, liars, thieves, cheaters, tax collectors, and soldiers. God has forgiven all sorts of people who have done a lot worse things than you. God will forgive anyone who comes to God with a contrite and repentant heart.

God expects us to recognize our sins and the commandments we have broken. God expects us to ask forgiveness for those things we have done wrong. God expects us to make right those things we have done wrong and then God expects us to go on. Dwelling on what we have done wrong does not fix the problem. We have actions we can take to move on from those things we have done wrong and then *vow not to do again*. That is the cycle of repentance and reconciliation with God.

Even if you screw up with the same thing again, God will still forgive you and love you. God has assured us through Jesus Christ that we all have a place in God's kingdom if we believe and have faith. God's grace will save us every time we screw up, no matter how many times, and no matter how many commandments we have broken, if we come back to God with a willing heart.

God has not forsaken you and God will always love you. Please believe that there is a place for *you* within God's kingdom and God wants you there more than anything.

THINGS TO THINK ABOUT

1. Do I believe God can forgive me?

2. Is there is a place for me in God's kingdom?

3. What do I need to do to come before God with a contrite heart?

DAY 34 Steps taken: _____ Miles journeyed: _____

Exercise chosen: _____

What I told God today: _____

_____

_____

_____

_____

Something I thought about: _____

_____

_____

_____

_____

Church is Boring

BIBLICAL BIG IDEA #35
Watch yourselves and the whole flock, in which the Holy Spirit has placed you as supervisors, to shepherd God's church, which he obtained with the death of his own Son. —Acts 20:28

Church can feel boring. Do you hear the "blah, blah, blah" of adults speaking throughout the service? Do you hear the words? Church is less boring the more you *participate* and engage in what is going on around you, rather than sit back and hear "blah, blah, blah."

There is no reason you cannot begin to pay attention and be involved in the different parts of the service, even though it may feel like the service is for adults only. As soon as you can read, you can sing the hymns and read the Bible passages. As soon as you can practice the discipline of focus and attention, you can listen to the sermon and think about how it applies to *your* life.

As soon as you acknowledge God in your life, you become responsible for building that love for God through activities at church. This will make the boredom go away. Having a relationship with someone takes work. It takes participation. It takes being involved in the relationship and honoring the sacrifice of what is given to *you*. It takes two to build a relationship and that includes your own action and participation.

God is calling you right now. You have a purpose, a reason, and a mission to make the world a better place. Part of going to church and participating in worship is building that relationship with God so you can hear that calling in your life. The more often you do something, the more it becomes a part of who you are. The more often you go to worship and make the activities in church a part of your everyday life, the less it will seem boring and more like how you are supposed to live. With every step you have taken in Christ Walk these forty days, you have taken a step in building your relationship with God. Each time you look at your step counter it can serve as a reminder of how far you have come in building that relationship.

THINGS TO THINK ABOUT

1. What parts of church do I think are boring?

2. What are some things I can do to make church less boring?

3. What are some things I have learned in church that I've applied in my everyday life?

DAY 35 Steps taken: _____ Miles journeyed: _____

Exercise chosen: _____

What I told God today: _____

_____

_____

_____

_____

Something I thought about: _____

_____

_____

_____

_____

I'm Too Old for Sunday School

BIBLICAL BIG IDEA #36

Teach them to your children, by talking about them when you are sitting around your house and when you are out and about, when you are lying down and when you are getting up.
—Deuteronomy 11:19

Much like going to church, going to Sunday school is how we learn about building our relationship with God. We cannot begin to understand our place in God's world without understanding the history of God's people over time in the world. The stories in the Bible teach us how people in history have had a relationship with God. Those stories also teach us how people have messed up their relationship with God.

Humans are flawed. No one is perfect. We need these teachings to understand how we are supposed to treat each other, how to live a holy life, how to take care of our bodies, how to honor God with our bodies.

Going to Sunday school teaches us these lessons and shows how the Bible stories fit into the context of our own life. Going to Sunday school does not have an age limit. Adults should not stop going to Sunday school and neither should you.

We like to think we know it all when it comes to God. We think that if we just love one another and be kind that is all there is to it. If there is one thing I've learned, it is that we will all be challenged with events in life that call into question things we've been taught or what would be the right way to respond in a situation. Life is not black and white. Going to Sunday school just equips you with more knowledge to help you make the right life decisions.

You are never too old for Sunday school.

THINGS TO THINK ABOUT

1. Do I feel like I am too old for Sunday school?

2. Is there something I can do, or a different class I can try?

3. What can I say to my Sunday school teacher about making class more applicable to my age group?

4. What do *I* want to get out of Sunday school?

DAY 36 Steps taken: _____ Miles journeyed: _____

Exercise chosen: _____

What I told God today: _____

_____

_____

_____

_____

Something I thought about: _____

_____

_____

_____

_____

37 Bullies

BIBLICAL BIG IDEA #37

Because he is praiseworthy, I cried out to the LORD, and I was saved from my enemies. —Psalm 18:3

Bullying is a hot topic at schools now. I am sure you had to sign an "anti-bullying" pledge of some sort during the school year. It is certainly sad that we have to sign an agreement to be kind to one another.

Bullying is not a Christian principle. We have discussed turning the other cheek when people are cruel to you. We have talked about loving your neighbor as yourself. We have reflected on kindness. We have discussed being the love of God in the world around us.

Bullying has no place in God's vision for us. If you yourself have been a bully, think of what you can do to make it right. Remember, it costs *nothing* to ask for forgiveness.

If *you* are being bullied, you need to get help. You can ask a trusted adult for advice. You can talk to your priest or pastor. You *can* talk to your parents. You can talk to a guidance counselor or a favorite teacher. You need to find someone to help you.

What does bullying really do? Bullying tears down the walls of who we think we are and damages our self-worth. It causes us to think we do not have a place in this world and strips us of a sense of purpose. Bullying causes us to question why we are here. Bullying can lead to thoughts of suicide because you may think you are not worth being a part of this world.

We are *all* different. There is no perfect child, or perfect teen, or perfect adult. Beauty comes in all sorts of shapes, sizes, ages, genders, and backgrounds. Each one of us brings unique talents to the table that the world needs. We all have different interests and strengths and we all have a purpose in God's eyes for being a part of this world. We need you here. Bullying is not the answer. Suicide is not the answer. Harming yourself or others is not the answer. Put your faith in God and an adult you trust and find a way to find your own self-purpose. Do not be a bully and do not let a bully strip you of who you are.

THINGS TO THINK ABOUT

1. Have I ever bullied someone? How did that make me feel?

2. Have I been or am I being bullied? How did that make me feel?

3. How is being different such a bad thing? A good thing?

DAY 37 Steps taken: _____ Miles journeyed: _____

Exercise chosen: _____

What I told God today: _____

_____

_____

_____

_____

Something I thought about: _____

_____

_____

_____

_____

DAY 38
Money, Money, Money

BIBLICAL BIG IDEA #38
Where your treasure is, there your heart will be also.
—Matthew 6:21

We live in a very materialistic society. We all like, want, and need things, which is why we often focus on how much money we have or don't have. Money is not bad. When you work hard, compensation often comes through money. However, money should not be the driver of our work. Remember, we are here for God and to do God's work in the world. You have a part in that purpose.

Money is often the way we support improvement in our church and community. As members of a church, we are called to tithe (or give 10 percent) of what we have to the church for it to support its mission in the world. The church is not a business. It cannot thrive without the financial support of its members. You are a part of that support.

The best advice I ever received when it came to giving to the church was to write that check to the church first thing each month—before I paid for anything else. I don't look at the bottom line of what I have, I give first and no matter how financially tight a month may be, somehow, God always manages to make it stretch when we give our first fruits to God.

God does not ask for a specific 10 percent from us. He asks for the best from us. He is asking for our time, money, talents, and heart for the world we live in today. Money is a part of the world we live in today. The giving of our money to God ensures that God is a part of how we want that world to work. You will get money when you work hard, but you will get so much more if you work hard for God.

THINGS TO THINK ABOUT

1. What do I want to work for?

2. Do I like money?

3. What would I like to do with that money?

DAY 38 Steps taken: _____   Miles journeyed: _____

Exercise chosen: _____

What I told God today: _____

_____

_____

_____

_____

Something I thought about: _____

_____

_____

_____

_____

39 How We Live This Life Matters

BIBLICAL BIG IDEA #39

But nobody knows when that day or hour will come, not the heavenly angels and not the Son. Only the Father knows.
—Matthew 24:36

I have recently concluded that we do not think enough about heaven. We do not live as though we were trying to get into heaven. Heaven is such a surreal time-place-event continuum, as we find so many of our worldly desires here on earth. We often cannot think of heaven until an event occurs that makes us question the importance of those earthly desires.

How we live our lives today, and the choices we make, impact every aspect of our long-term relationships with God. The daily choices we make shape the lives we are building. The lives we build help us to face the events that make us question everything. If you have not begun to question, you will. It is fine to have questions about your spirituality and God. Just make sure God is a part of the questioning process.

This all matters because there is life after death. There is a heaven with angels, archangels, and all the company of heaven. In heaven there is God, with peace, and no more suffering. Jesus has promised us this if we believe. This means that at some point, our sufferings on earth will no longer matter, or hurt, or cause us sadness. We will be one with God and everything will be all right.

As we wait for this time with God, God does call us to work in the world to make it a better place. We are here to care for those on our earthly home as they wait for *their* time to go heaven. We are here to spread the word of God and God's love so that no one is left out of this chance for heaven. We are here to use our bodies in order to love with our whole selves and to give ourselves to others, just as Jesus gave his life for us.

Your life on earth matters to the life you will have in heaven.

THINGS TO THINK ABOUT

1. What do I think about heaven?

2. How am I living my life now with the goal of going to heaven?

3. Why do I think I am here?

DAY 39 Steps taken: _____ Miles journeyed: _____

Exercise chosen: _____

What I told God today: _____

_____

_____

_____

_____

Something I thought about: _____

_____

_____

_____

_____

40 What Now?

BIBLICAL BIG IDEA #40

*I thank my God every time I mention you in my prayers. I'm
thankful for all of you every time I pray, and it is always a prayer
full of joy. I'm glad because of the way you have been my
partners in the ministry of the gospel from the time you first
believed it until now. I'm sure about this: the one who started
a good work in you will stay with you to complete the job by
the day of Christ Jesus.* —Philippians 1:3–6

You have come on this journey for forty days with me. I hope that you
have walked and talked the Christ Walk way. I hope that you have come
to a deeper understanding of God, and your place in God's world. I hope
that you have built some healthy habits that you will use to build a stronger, healthier you to continue God's work in the world.

What do we do now? Keep walking. Keep talking. The journey does
not end here. This is a lifelong journey that does not end. I am still walking my Christ Walk journey. Each day I learn something new about God's
purpose for me. We keep working every day for a better world. We keep
working every day to show God's love. We keep working every day on the
purpose that God has for us. We will often stumble. Sometimes we will
fall, but the most important part is to keep going.

It is not over yet.

THINGS TO THINK ABOUT

1. What have I learned these past forty days?

2. How can I continue my Christ Walk journey?

3. Who can I take with me on my next Christ Walk journey?

DAY 40   Steps taken: _____   Miles journeyed: _____

Exercise chosen: _____

What I told God today: _____

_____

_____

_____

_____

Something I thought about: _____

_____

_____

_____

_____

Conclusion

Congratulations! You have finished the Christ Walk Kids forty-day spiritual fitness program!

Keep moving. The journey does not end here. You have many steps ahead of you on your path, so keep moving and living a Christ-centered life. If you want to keep in touch with me on your journey, be sure to follow me on social media:

Blog: www.christwalk40day.blogspot.com

Twitter: @christwalk1

Facebook: www.facebook.com/Christwalk40day

Instagram: @christwalk1

Just to show yourself how far you went, take a moment to count up your journey over the last forty days.

DURING THE PAST FORTY DAYS I:

Walked this number of total steps: _____

Walked this number of total miles: _____

Learned this Biblical Big Idea: _____

_____

_____

_____

_____

Learned this about myself: _____

_____

_____

_____

_____

Way to go! It's been a pleasure sharing this journey with you. Keep going!

In Christ,
—Anna

APPENDIX A

Suggested Walking Routes*

Individual and Beginner Routes

Name of Route	Description	Total Distance	Distance Per Day
Nazareth Challenge	The route between Jesus' hometown of Nazareth and Jerusalem	65 miles	1.6 miles or 4,000 steps per day
Jerusalem to Damascus	Paul's conversion on the Damascus Road took place along this journey.	150 miles	3.75 miles or 7,500 steps per day

Intermediate Routes

Name of Route	Description	Total Distance	Distance Per Day
The Jerusalem Challenge	The *Via Dolorosa* (Way of Sorrows) is the route Jesus took through Jerusalem during the last week of his life, which included his preaching in the Temple, clearing the Temple of the money-changers, his Last Supper with the disciples, his arrest in the Garden of Gethsemane, his trial, and his crucifixion.	88 miles	2.2 miles or about 5,500 steps per day
Damascus to Caesarea	One of Paul's missionary journeys	200 miles	5 miles or 10,000 steps per day (a pedometer is recommended)

*All distances are approximate and renditions from maps of the Holy Land.

Advanced

Name of Route	Description	Total Distance	Distance Per Day
The Bethlehem Challenge	The distance between Bethlehem and Jerusalem, representing the beginning and end of Christ's life	200 miles	5 miles or 10,000 steps per day (without using a pedometer)*

*This challenge is done without a pedometer. This means that you will get 5 miles of exercise during one workout instead of accumulating the miles over the course of a day with a pedometer.

Name of Route	Description	Total Distance	Distance Per Day
Tarsus to Jerusalem Challenge	One of Paul's missionary journeys	390 miles	9.75 miles of 19,500 steps per day (pedometer recommended)
The Exodus Challenge	The route the Israelites traveled to get to the Promised Land of Canaan	375 miles	9.4 miles or 18,750 steps per day (pedometer recommended)

Group Challenges

Pool each individual participant's miles each week to reach a group distance goal.

Name of Route	Description	Total Distance	Distance Per Day
The Abraham Migration	Represents Abraham's wanderings to find the Promised Land to begin the birth of God's people	900 miles	22.5 miles per day
Jerusalem to Antioch (round trip)	One of Paul's missionary journeys	705 miles	17.25 miles per day
Paul's First Missionary Journey	Paul's first mission trip	1,300 miles	32.5 miles per day
Ephesus to Jerusalem	One of Paul's missionary trips	800 miles	20 miles per day
Jerusalem to Rome	The end of the road for Paul	1,800 miles	45 miles per day

Group Challenges (continued)

Name of Route	Description	Total Distance	Distance Per Day
Jerusalem to Corinth	One of Paul's missionary journeys	1,050 miles	26.25 miles per day
Antioch to Philippi	A portion of Paul's third missionary journey	950 miles	23.75 miles per day

Beginner Walks

Nazareth Challenge: It is 65 miles between Jesus' hometown of Nazareth and Jerusalem. This is approximately 1.6 miles each day for forty days to walk the distance of the route that Jesus preached to reach his end in Jerusalem. Set a goal to walk 1.6 miles each day or 4,000 steps per day during Lent (or any forty day period of your choosing), or complete 65 miles by the end of the six-week period.

Jerusalem to Damascus: This journey represents Paul's conversion on the Damascus Road. It is 150 miles or 3.75 miles per day or 7,500 steps a day.

Intermediate Walks

Jerusalem Challenge: During Jesus' final days, his route through Jerusalem included preaching at the Temple, clearing the Temple of the money changers, the last supper with his disciples, his arrest in the Garden of Gethsemane, his trial, Peter's denial, and his crucifixion. This route was approximately 2.2 miles in length. Set a goal to walk 2.2 miles each day during Lent, or about 5,500 steps per day.

Damascus to Caesarea: One of Paul's missionary journeys was about 200 miles or 5 miles per day or 10,000 steps a day. You can use a pedometer throughout the day to accumulate the miles.

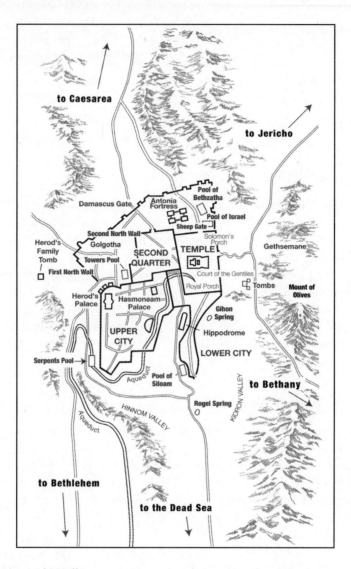

to Caesarea

to Jericho

Pool of
Bethzatha

Damascus Gate   Antonia
Fortress

Pool of Israel

Sheep Gate

Second North Wall   Solomon's
Porch

Herod's   Golgotha   TEMPLE   Gethsemane
Family   SECOND
Tomb   Towers Pool   QUARTER

First North Wall   Court of the Gentiles

Royal Porch   Tombs   Mount of
Herod's   Hasmoneam   Olives
Palace   Palace
Gihon
Spring

UPPER   Hippodrome
CITY

LOWER CITY

Serpents Pool

Pool of
Aqueduct   Siloam   to Bethany

Rogel Spring
HINNOM VALLEY

Aqueduct

to Bethlehem

to the Dead Sea

Advanced Walks

Bethlehem Challenge: It is five miles between Bethlehem and Jerusalem. This represents the beginning to the end of Christ's journey. Set a
goal to walk five miles without using a pedometer.

Tarsus to Jerusalem: This is Paul's route from his home town of Tarsus
to Jerusalem. I look at this journey as a reflection of where we started in
life and what draws us on our calling with Christ. 390 miles or 9.75 miles
a day or 19,500 steps a day

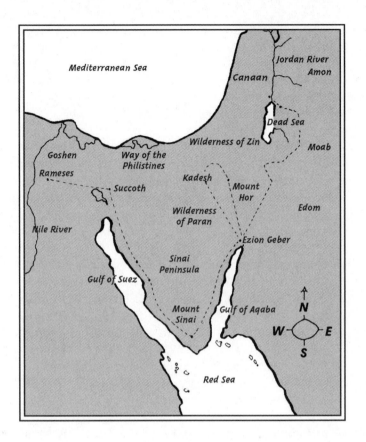

The Exodus: The route the Israelites traveled to get to the Promised Land is 375 miles, 9.4 miles per day or 18,750 steps per day. (This may be used as a group challenge.)

Group Challenges

These goals should be divided based on the number of people in your group and how many miles each group member will commit to walking during the forty-day challenge:

The Abraham Migration: This represents Abraham's wanderings to find the Promised Land to begin the birth of God's people. It is roughly 900 miles, or 22.5 miles a day.

Jerusalem to Antioch: This is the first part of Paul's second missionary journey. Paul was preaching to the Gentiles in Antioch. This was one of the first times in which God's word was shared to other Christians not of Jewish descent. This is a round trip of 705 miles or 17.25 miles a day.

Antioch to Cyprus: This is part of Paul's 1st missionary journey. Paul and Barnabas travel from Antioch to Barnabas' home in Salamis, Cyprus to preach the word of God. 1,300 miles or 32.5 miles a day

Ephesus to Jerusalem: This is a portion of Paul's third missionary journey. The Letter to the Ephesians is one of Paul's most famous letters written while building the church in the city of Ephesus. The church later became one of the heads of the seven churches of Asia Minor and contributed to the spread of Christianity across what is modern day Turkey. 800 miles or 20 miles a day

Paul's Journey to Rome: Paul's journey from Jerusalem to Rome where he finally died for his beliefs. It is said that Paul's body is buried underneath St. Paul's Cathedral in Vatican City. 1,800 miles or 45 miles a day

Jerusalem to Corinth: The full route of Paul's third missionary journey to Corinth, Greece. Paul is the founder of the Christian church in Corinth. In his letter to the Corinthians, Paul gives thanks for his health, his journey, his deliverance from dangers, and for the people of Corinth. 1050 miles or 26.25 miles a day

Antioch to Philippi: This is a portion of Paul's 3rd Missionary Journey. The church in Philippi is the first Christian church founded by Paul in Europe. 950 miles or 23.75 miles a day

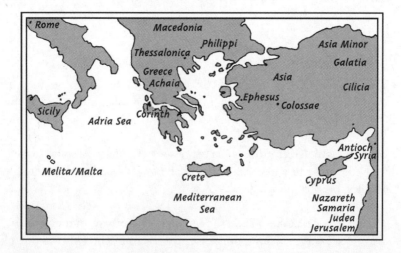

Pedometer Usage and Mileage Calculations

You can purchase a pedometer from any sporting or general goods store. When you clip your pedometer onto your waistband, it should be at about the height of your hipbone. Roughly 2,000 steps equal a mile, but steps and mileage calculation depend on the length of your stride. For the ease of calculation you can use 2,000 steps to a mile, or measure your stride and have the pedometer calculate it for you. You do not have to walk; you can use a treadmill, run, bike, swim or whatever activity you choose to do. Approximately fifteen minutes of physical activity will equal a mile if you are unable to calculate the mileage. (For example, fifteen minutes of an aerobics/yoga class would be a mile for the purpose of this program.)

If you are unable to exercise, consider using each fifteen-minute block in volunteering or in prayer. Our goal is to transform spiritually as well as physically. There are no penalties in Christ Walk! Focus on things you can do to change your life through increased activity, or increased prayer, or increased work for others. Use your pedometer all day so that *all* of your activity will be included towards your goal. Please join us in a journey taking a step of faith in Christ.

Mileage Calculation Chart

Activity	Time	Steps	Record Miles As:
Walking	15–20 minutes	2,000–2,500	1 or distance on route
Running	Varies	2,000–2,500	Check route distance
Biking	Varies	N/A	Check odometer distance
Aerobics	15 minutes	Varies	1
Dancing	15 minutes	Varies	1
Yoga	15 minutes	Varies	1
Prayer/Meditation	15 minutes	Varies	1
Volunteerism	15 minutes	Varies	1

Agenda for a Christ Walk Kids Group

Start off with an icebreaker. Find someone in your group you do not know and introduce yourself, telling them something unique about you. Keep talking and asking questions until you figure out what you have in common. Once you know what you have in common, find a group of two and repeat the exercise until the four of you have something in common. Repeat this process until the group is complete and the whole group has discovered something that they have in common. (It cannot be church or Christ Walk.)

When the icebreaker is complete, you can then work as a group to come up with:

- A team name;
- A team prayer—write it as a group;
- Your team's walking/mileage goal;
- Your individual walking/running/biking goal;
- Something that you would like to raise money for by completing that goal (a mission you would like to support) and how to do it.

Consider finding a fun walk/run to do together as a team towards the end of Lent—not mandatory, just an idea for fundraising. People could sponsor you a dollar a mile, or something for completing the race or completing your mileage journey. Or you can donate the money raised to the church's mission fund. If you would like, each of you can share what you learned. If your church also has an adult Christ Walk group, talk with them about your accomplishments.

Suggestions for Groups

Christ Walk was intended to be a group activity. People who have communities of fitness or teams of fitness are more likely to be successful in their goals. Teams are successful when they:

- Meet together;
- Exercise together;
- Pray together;
- Share successes and challenges together;
- Encourage each other.

If you are not experiencing Christ Walk as a part of a church educational or devotional period, try to get a group of friends together to experience the lessons and activities together. Your Bible study, men's, or women's group can complete Christ Walk. The purpose is to commit to improving your health together as you help each other along to a healthier you. If you do not have access to a group, join a virtual team through Fitbit, Facebook, or another group so that you are not alone in your journey.

Christ Walk can be found online at:

- Facebook: www.facebook.com/christwalk40day ;
- Twitter: @christwalk1;
- Blog: www.blogspot.christwalk40day.com .

Another suggestion for groups is to invite a fitness professional to discuss principles of fitness as a special guest. I also recommend that a fitness professional come to conduct fitness testing with each individual followed by individualized fitness plan recommendations based on the results of the fitness test for everyone.

Suggestions for Group Leaders

If you are taking on the role as a Christ Walk group leader, congratulations! What an awesome experience for you and your team or church. You can join the Christ Walk forum on Facebook to discuss ideas and goals with members of the Christ Walk community around the globe! I am happy to provide feedback or guidance on running a group Christ Walk. Christ Walk can be found online at:

- Facebook: www.facebook.com/christwalk40day
- Twitter: @christwalk1
- Blog: www.blogspot.christwalk40day.com

The number one guidance I offer in leading Christ Walk is to give freely of yourself and your experience. You may have a lot of fitness experience or none at all, but since we all have health, we all have a perspective that can be shared and discussed in our small-group settings that are valuable to anyone in the room. I have led groups from as few as five participants to as many as eighty, and the experience can be as much as we choose to share with each other during our time together. Give freely of yourself and your experience. This builds a bond of a shared experience.

There are several ways that the Christ Walk experience can be structured for groups:

- As a simple Bible study, meet each week to discuss the "Thoughts to Ponder" after each day's reading. Simply share your experiences with those meditations. Make sure that everyone reports and tracks their miles to their destination.
- Meet each week to focus on a different topic (See Appendix G for an outline):
  - Week One: Introduction
  - Week Two: Physical Health
  - Week Three: Mental Health
  - Week Four: Spiritual Health

- Week Five: Nutrition
- Week Six: Pot Luck and Graduation/Sharing

• Meet each week to discuss one of the scripture readings from the meditations, sharing what each says to the members of your group about their health.
  - Week One: Introduction
  - Week Two: Yoga
  - Week Three: Aerobics
  - Week Four: Guided Walk
  - Week Five: Weight Lifting
  - Week Six: Meditation

• Meet each week and have a theological reflection on one of the topics on the week's readings. Discuss the topic from the point of view of creation, sin, judgment, repentance, and redemption. (See Appendix G for an outline.)
  - Week One: Introduction
  - Week Two: Creation—How is God creating something new in us?
  - Week Three: Sin—Where have we gone wrong?
  - Week Four: Judgment—Where are we caught up short?
  - Week Five: Repentance—Where have we sought forgiveness?
  - Week Six: Redemption—Where have we been forgiven?

• Meet each week and provide keys to healthy living.
  - Week One: Introduction
  - Week Two: Health Fair/Health Assessment
  - Week Three: Making Change/Change Exercise/Goal Setting
  - Week Four: Fitness Testing
  - Week Five: Cooking Classes
  - Week Six: Healthy Potluck

Need other Ideas? Join me on Facebook, Twitter, or the blog for a discussion of group options. I am happy to answer questions as they are posted!

Happy Christ Walking!

Steps and Mileage Tracker

You can use the following space to track your progress through your challenge. Each day, add in your steps for the day, the miles for the day, and then add that into the total column for a running total of your progress. You can also make copies of these pages to use in subsequent challenges! Enjoy your journey!

Date	Steps	Miles	Today's Total	Running Total

Date	Steps	Miles	Today's Total	Running Total

Date	Steps	Miles	Today's Total	Running Total

Acknowledgments

Wow. No one goes on a journey alone. I have never been alone on my Christ Walk journeys, either the one for adults and now the one for our precious youth. You all are the future of the church. First, I want to thank my kids; there were times they were probably ignored more than they should have been while I wrote. This book is for you, Merryn and Patton. It covers almost everything I want you to think about while growing up as a child of God. Mama loves you. So does God.

To my editor, Sharon: You trusted me again with another book. Wow. I am still reeling from the first go-round. Three is the charm?

To my friends and family. To my Groots. For my mama who never stopped believing in me even when I was struggling to find my own way as a kid.

To my husband, Treb: Wow, "thanks" is not enough. You are an amazing father. I certainly could not have done this without you. Thank you for teaching me every day to be a better parent and for all your unofficial editing duties. My journey would be ever so lonely without you. Let's keep walking together. I'm told the best is yet to be.

And God. Thank you. You are good.